Thank You God, Jennifer, Makenzie, Family, Friends, Life and Others who have helped me understand how important it is to win moments!

WINNING MOMENTS

The Quest for the 24 Hour Workout
How to turn EVERYTHING we do into better health
John Fresh, D.C.

Table of Contents:

Introduction

Always get in a good posture and engage the core before moving your body. This will protect the spine, create a power posture, and strengthen muscles.

This book is designed to bring awareness to all the moments that make up our day and how they are an opportunity to create a better healthier more active life. The idea of winning moments began, first, with me having to find less painful ways to brush my teeth, walk, sit, sleep, cough, sneeze, get dressed, everything, because I was living with excruciating pain. Later as a chiropractor, practically everyday, I would hear, and still hear, about how people injure themselves doing normal everyday stuff. When I would ask people how they were performing their daily activities I realized that people were not taught how to care for their neck and back as they go throughout their day. The truth is, I was not taught either, however, my suffering forced me to learn. I would say learn quickly, but I have been working on winning daily moments for over 20 years. In the beginning, I was learning how to avoid pain, today I am performing these same activities as a way to improve posture, strength, flexibility, endurance, and balance. Winning moments can take your health anywhere you want it to go. Many people wait until it is time to exercise to take care of themselves. Instead, what I have learned from pain, discomfort, tightness,...and especially chiropractic, as my teacher, is how to do every activity we ask our body to perform each day, in a way that builds a healthier spine, and ultimately a healthier life. This is done by utilizing the same activities we do every day, over and over, that cause many people stress, strain, and injury. Slight modifications and focus on how we carry and move our body in these moments that make up a day can turn daily activities into better health. This book includes everything from going to bed, sleeping, getting up from bed, going to the bathroom, brushing teeth, getting dressed, exercising, getting in the shower, sitting, driving, working, playing with the kids, watching tv, reading, to preparing for bed the next day, and everything in between. I try to win moments when sleeping, awake, at work, home, doing yard work, emptying the dishwasher, taking out the trash, running errands like food shopping, including how I carry bags into the house. I try to have this winning moments awareness with everything I do and everywhere I go. I am always looking for better ways to reduce stress and promote health in my spine and body with every activity I perform. My ultimate goal is winning every possible moment of my day in the quest for the 24-hour workout.

My goal with this book is to help you win one moment in your day and experience the change it makes in your life.

There are two ways we can look at our day and how we're having an impact on our health. One is through a microscope, how we're feeling each moment and what we are doing each moment. Two is through a telescope, how our daily decisions and choices affect our health over the weeks, months, and years to come. The telescope helps us minimize negative thoughts and habits about how we feel or what we feel like doing right now and gives us the proper motivation concerning the type of life we want to live, the level of health we want to have, and the daily habits required to live that life. Now, the benefit of the microscope perspective is that if we have the right focus and we are doing the right things each moment we will give ourselves the best chance possible to have an active healthy life now and in the future.

Remember, how we feel today is the result of choices we have made weeks or months ago. How we choose to live today will determine how we feel weeks and months from now. Change happens with consistency and time.

The good news is that while following this book it won't add one minute to your day. It follows everything we already do in a day and how to perform those activities as exercises we would do at a gym or at home to get a stronger spine and body. Many times we go through our day in a way that causes unnecessary stress. This stress will break down our body and health. When our health gets bad enough we spend all our time and money trying to get our health back. We still don't make it easy on ourselves because in addition to neglecting our health, we still need to overcome excuses like we don't have time and we are too busy to take care of ourselves. Comments like these lead to more problems every time. What if instead of those moments that cause unnecessary stress, injury, and pain to our body, we repurpose them into winning moments. Moments that produce the health and ability to live the life of our dreams year after year.

Health is one of the most important things to everyone. If we are investing 2 hours out of 24 hours in a day and seeing amazing results to our health and in our lives, imagine what 10 or, if possible, 24 hours of investing in your health could do. I'm so grateful that when we invest in our health for 2 hours, 8%, or 1 hour, 4%, or just 30 minutes, 2% of our day, that our body is able to improve our health, it's truly incredible. What an amazing body. This is in spite of the fact that we may not have been taught the proper way to perform daily habits or have picked up poor habits that have a negative effect on our health for the next 22 hours or 92% of our day. The only other time we may think about our health is deciding what we are going to eat. This can be especially true when we are feeling good and there are no aches or pain to remind us that everything we do in our day matters. The time you put aside to invest in your health is very valuable, but it only minimizes or delays you feeling the damage caused by poor daily habits, it is a losing battle. However, the more moments you win in a day the further those benefits will go. It's threefold one, your time investing in yourself will go further. When you have less stress to take off the body, your body will invest more of that time into building higher levels of health. Two, you are not only reducing stress on the body by winning more moments, but you are also limiting the negative effects, that accumulating stress can have over time. Third, you are now actually promoting health throughout your day, by increasing the time you invest in yourself by 50, 60, 70, 80, or even 90%.

Percent of time in a day(estimates):
Sleep: avg 6-8 hours, 30%
Getting Up/Getting Ready/Breakfast/Exercise: avg 2-3 hours, 10%
Drive Time/Running Errands/House Work/Work: avg 9-11 hours, 40%
Practices/Games/Dinner/Home: avg 4-5 hours, 20 %

Two key areas that we need to be aware of to achieve the health we desire, to live the life of our dreams. One is our ability to reduce the amount of unnecessary stress on our body mentally, physically, and emotionally. Two is the time we spend investing in our health each day mentally, physically, and emotionally. The more we reduce unnecessary stress and the more we invest in ourselves the quicker and more efficiently our health will improve.

One powerful way to improve health is created by winning moments. Take sitting for example, here is an activity that has been shown to decrease quality of life, shorten lifespan, and can cause neck, back, and sciatica pain. That seems like a significant amount of unnecessary stress to me. But what if we could take that same activity and instead of it causing unnecessary stress, we can win that moment by improving posture, balance, and core strength with a couple minor adjustments to how we are sitting. Winning moments can be anything from being able to perform a simple activity like putting on your shoes with less pain, to performing deep stretches while putting on your shoes. This book is about how you can be winning moments in your life.

Our ultimate goal in winning moments is the quest for the 24-hour workout. We can at least try to perform everything we do with awareness, intention and focus on building a power posture and active life that produces strength, flexibility, endurance, and balance.

The three keys to winning moments are awareness, a power posture, and muscle engagement.

The first level is being aware. Utilizing cues or reminders can help us focus on our intention to win moments. Examples of cues or reminders to win moments could be wearing a rubber band around our wrist, a sticky note to yourself on a bathroom mirror, in the car, or on the computer. A great cue for a power posture is to set up a computer screen, pad, or phone so that the screen is difficult to see when you are in a poor posture When the screen becomes difficult to see, don't adjust your screen, adjust your posture. You can even play a game like how many times do you need to adjust your posture in a week. Try and get a lower score each week. In a car, this is great to do with the rear view mirror. When you slouch you can't see the entire rear window, don't adjust the mirror, the mirror is adjusted for a power posture. Adjust your back to a power posture, you'll know when you are in a power posture because you'll be able to see perfectly out the rear window. These are a few of many types of examples of how cues contribute to awareness and ultimately winning moments.

The second level is having a power posture in those moments to maximize spinal health, nerve flow and life to the muscles, tissues, and cells of our body. Power postures are postures we use, during any and all activities, that protects our spine the most, while positioning our muscles to be used where they are the strongest. The third level is core and muscle engagement. Every muscle working together to create a power posture, strength, flexibility, endurance, and balance. This applies to everything we do including walking, sitting, exercising, cleaning, getting dressed, getting in and out of the car,...anything that involves moving our body or holding it in any position as we go throughout our day. That means everything, everywhere, at all times. We also want to make sure we are not overworking one side of our body more than the other, we should try to do what we can to work the right and left sides of our body equally.

A lot of people's health issues, not just musculoskeletal issues, are because of poor health in that person's hard and soft tissues. Hard and Soft Tissue Work go great together. Hard tissue are the bones of your spine and posture. Soft tissue are the discs in between the bones, the ligaments that hold the bones together, the tendons that attach the muscles to the bones, and the fascia, which is a stiffer less flexible type of soft tissue that wraps around everything inside your body, including your brain, and is in between your muscles.

Think of a telephone pole and the cables that hold it and balance it. If you only work on soft tissue, which represents the cables, they will be under more stress and wear down faster with a pole, hard tissue, that is not balanced, tilted, or leaning to one side, which represents poor posture or subluxation, a joint in the spine that is not moving properly or stuck in a bad position.

If the posture or pole in this analogy has gotten stuck in a position that causes the cables or muscles more stress, it would be important to unlock that pole or posture for better alignment. This will allow the cables or muscle to be under less stress and better balanced.
Equally important is that the cable or muscles don't negatively influence the pole or posture. An imbalance, tightness in muscles or fascia, trigger points, scar tissue, or poor daily habits can negatively affect the pole, meaning your posture and spine.

If it helps you can also think of the Leaning Tower of Pisa, how much more stress is on the materials and how often do they have to work on those materials to keep that structure standing versus a structure that has good alignment. The one additional thing we need to consider when talking about our body is the importance of flexibility, mobility, and balance. Mobility is what makes our body so great and where a lot of our problems can originate. It's so important that we're taking care of both our hard and soft tissue each day because if one is working and moving well and the other isn't, both will negatively be affected. However, if we are investing time towards our hard and soft tissue, when both are working and moving well you'll feel better and have a much more active life than if you were only caring for one or the other.

Hard and soft tissue both, as well as many other areas of health, need to be addressed for you to experience the best that your body has to offer.

Any one thing is NOT the only thing a body needs to be at its' best.

Here is a sample of what a day of winning moments may look like in our quest for the 24-hour workout. Even though our day may vary based on our job or responsibilities these concepts can apply or adapt to any lifestyle or schedule. It's a way of thinking about how we do everything we need to do.

Each moment we perform an activity and how we perform that activity will leave a positive or negative residue on the next moment or activity. We want to win as many moments as we can to do our part in creating positive MOMENTum.

This is NOT medical advice, because I don't know what you are going through right now and more importantly why. These type of questions can only be answered by a thorough examination and proper diagnosis. **My first recommendation is to see the appropriate health care provider.**

Chapter 1

HOURS 0-10

BEFORE BED/SLEEPING/GETTING UP/GETTING READY FOR THE DAY

BEFORE BED

Great news!!! Before the alarm rings in the morning we are already 9-10 hours into our workout, depending on how well and long we slept. So let's make sure we're making the most of our time asleep. The first thing is, *before we even go to bed*, begin to slow down the rush of thoughts from our day. Some people use a song or a landmark on the drive home as a cue to remind themselves to at least attempt to decompress and get ready to be present at home. Before we get home, once we get home, or before we go to bed we should relax and refocus with deep breathing, meditation, and my favorite, prayer. This also works great in the morning or anytime throughout the day.

Deep breathing, meditation, and prayer are like a superpower that can penetrate the greatest amount of stress and provide us with the strength we need to get through anything, even when we don't know how we are going to get through it.

We should also do light stretching to unwind areas of stress that have snuck their way into our body throughout the day before they negatively affect our health while we're sleeping. This is a pivotal winning moment because of the impact it has on how we will sleep that night!

The sooner we remove stress from our body the better the body can perform what it's naturally designed to do which is heal, repair, and provide us with what we need to have the best life possible....Health!

It is important right before you go to bed, or anytime, that you are being careful about what images, shows, sounds, or information you are allowing into your brain before you go to bed. That can be the information your brain focuses on and influence how well you sleep. There are many articles that talk about the negative effects of cellphone and other devices. The light and the EMF's (electromagnetic fields) emitted by electronic devices have a negative effect on rest and health. These devices include cell phones, routers, cordless phones, smart meters, baby monitors, and other wireless devices. If you would like more information about EMF's or other great information, Mercola.com is a great resource. If you can, meaning there are no emergencies or people that need to reach you, put your phone on airplane mode and keep it away from the bed. Keep a notepad and pen or pencil by the bed to jot down any thoughts, so your mind can rest easier.

SLEEPING

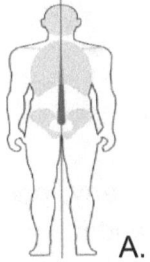
A.

When we lay down to sleep we want to lay in the same posture we would be in while standing in a power posture. A Power Posture is when looking at ourselves in a mirror(Image A), from the front view of ourselves, the middle of our forehead, nose, and chin should line up straight down the middle of our chest, and straight down between the middle of our legs.

When visualizing a power poster from the side(Image B), our ear should be over the middle of our shoulder, and our shoulder over the middle of our hips. Since our knees may be bent when we sleep they may not line up, but our hips should still line up with our ankles.

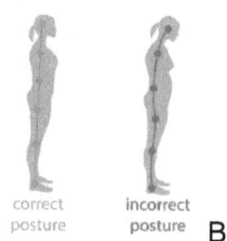

correct
posture

incorrect
posture   B.

We can use whatever pillows and positions necessary to achieve our power posture, use pillows to support our head and neck(Image C...This picture shows good alignment, but does not show the pillow supporting the neck, which I recommend), pillows to keep our arms supported(Image D), or pillows between our legs(Image E) to keep good hip alignment for side sleepers.

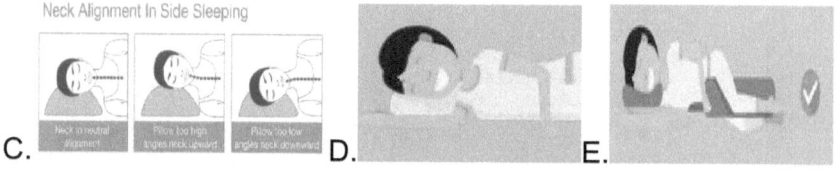

C.   D.   E.

Using pillows as supports for many people has reduced or eliminated headaches, neck, back, sciatica, and hip pain, it has even helped people who experience arm and hand pain, numbness, or tingling while they sleep. Back sleepers may want a pillow under their knees(Image F) to keep them slightly bent. All back sleepers should have a pillow(Image G) that keeps their neck in a good posture.

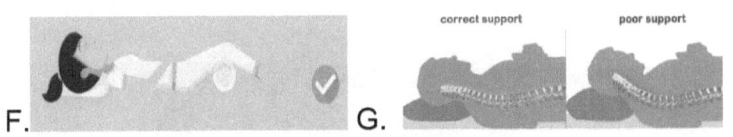

F.   G.

Every part of your body should be supported in a power posture by your pillow and mattress, with no spaces in between. If there are spaces that means your muscles will have to work harder and overtime a poor posture will develop from your body sagging to conform to the bed. If we have poor posture when we sleep, think of how it would feel, night after night, to have your head, neck, back or hips turned, tilted, or twisted for eight hours. This can help us realize how powerful sleep can be beyond just the rest we're getting and the repair that our body is doing. This is also a great time for us to do our cervical curve work(Image H). Either early in the morning or before we go to sleep while lying on our back on the bed or floor. Place a small foam roll, rolled up towel, or a small rounded pillow in the middle of the neck. Our head and shoulders will rest on the bed or floor, while the middle of our neck will be lifted up in an arc shape (think of what the curve of a bridge looks like) over the roll, towel, or pillow. Start out for a couple minutes at a time, working up each day to 15 minutes.

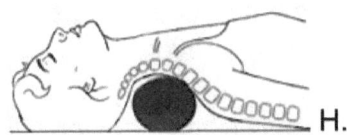

H.

It is vital that we reverse the damaging effects and loss of curve in our neck that occurs with computer work, reading, looking at our phone or other devices. This ultimately is one of the major causes of tech neck or poor posture. It happens from any neck and shoulder postures that cause us to look down, bringing our chin closer to our neck, or our head to move forward in front of our body, while our shoulders are rounded and slumped forward, for long periods of time. This poor posture will multiply the amount of stress on our entire spine(Image I).

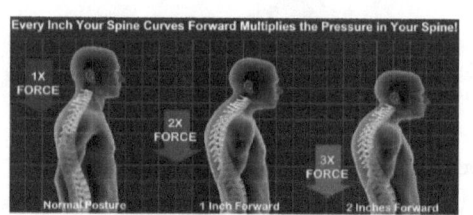

I.

Poor postures over time cause a straightening or even reversing of the curve in our neck. Losing our neck curve alone has been linked to many health issues that lead to a decreased quality of life. When our time is up from doing our neck curve work we need to use our hands to lift our head up off the roll, towel, or pillow. The neck muscles are very relaxed and stretched when we are doing our curve work, we want to give them an opportunity to reset before we ask our neck muscles to start working again.

We shouldn't be too hard on ourselves when considering sleeping. All we can do is start in the right posture and hope we sleep in that position longer and longer each night. The less stress we are under while sleeping, hopefully, the less we will move from our power posture. We also need to do our best to not use our head and neck to turn when we sleep, it can injure our neck trying to lift our body. It is better to use the hand of our top arm to push off the bed to help us turn or move.

A very common question I get is the *type of pillow or mattress* someone should be using. Everyone needs to be on the best possible pillow and mattress for them because of how important sleep is and how much time we spend sleeping. Here are some obvious signs that you are on the wrong pillow or mattress for you. You went to sleep feeling fine, but you wake up with headaches, neck, back, arm, or leg stiffness or pain. You wake up tired or feeling worse than when you went to bed. When people tell me they wake up with problems or wake up feeling worse, I know we need to address their pillow and mattress. My opinion is that it is very difficult to recommend one pillow or mattress that will be perfect for everyone. My first suggestion before you go out and buy anything is to talk to a chiropractor about the proper posture and support, for you, as you sleep. Earlier we had talked about the best postures to sleep in(Image J), however, some people have unique factors, like neck, shoulder, back, or hip problems that need to be taken into consideration when determining the best sleeping posture for them. It is important for you to know what position you should be in when sleeping. Next, experiment with what you have access to right at home. You can start with the proper sleeping posture while making sure you are supporting every part of your body as mentioned in the sleeping section above(Please review the power posture for sleeping and how to support your entire body).

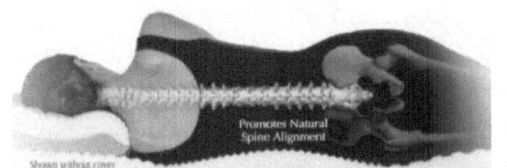

J.

When you get into your best posture take a *5-10 minute deep breath relaxation body scan test*. Scan your body as you are taking deep relaxing breaths. Make sure that each and every muscle is releasing and relaxing. Every part of your body should be supported by the pillow or mattress, your head, neck, the side of your body, your hips, everything. There should be no space between you and the pillow or mattress. This is a great test for pillows, mattresses, recliners, couches, anything you spend a good amount of time on each day. If your body is not passing the relaxation test than chances are that through the night those parts of your body are not getting the alignment, relaxation, and rest they need. This can be the reason you are waking up in the middle of the night in pain and the reason you are waking up in the morning tired, tight, or in pain.

Here are some more things you can do to find the right pillow and mattress for you. After you have tried all the pillows and mattresses in your house remember if there has been any pillow or mattress that you had gotten a good night's sleep on, like at a hotel, friend, or family members house. Find the name and characteristics of that pillow or mattress to get you started. If you feel your mattress is too soft, take off the pillow top or put a board in between the mattresses to make them more firm. If your mattress feels too firm, get a pillow or foam mattress topper to try something softer. When you go to a mattress store test each mattress in the position you sleep in and take the 5-10 minute deep breath relaxation body scan test. This will give you some of the best information you will need to pick the best pillow and mattress. I have a great story that illustrated how well this works. I had a patient come in while I was writing this book. They told me they got a mattress they love. I said, what did you do to find the perfect mattress, hoping to glean some additional insight. They said I did what you told me, I went into the mattress store, laid on the mattresses, took a couple of deep breathes and picked the one that felt the best, that supported me the most, and I felt the most relaxed. When I saw them again, I asked, how do you like the mattress, they said, it's great!

GETTING UP

Alarm clock rings, we jump out of bed! STOP! We hear so many people say their backs are tight and sore when they first get up in the morning and as the day goes on it loosens up. *So before we jump out of bed, let's not miss an opportunity to improve our health.* When we wake up it's a good idea to do a nice slow stretch, by reaching our hands over our head, stretching our feet and toes down, while giving our body an internal squeeze(Image K).

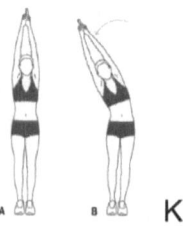

K.

It can also feel good while lying flat on our back with our feet together to let our knees fall away from each other, opening our hips, like a butterfly stretch(Image L). While in the butterfly stretch you can do gentle side stretches.

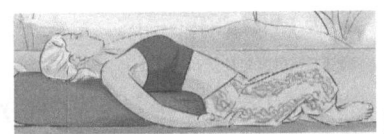

L.

Then we can pull one leg at a time into our chest, then both legs(Image M). While doing your first-morning stretch or stretching with your knees into your chest you can alternate flexing one foot at a time by pointing your toes. You can add flexing your feet to many leg, hip, or low back stretches. It is equally beneficial to add stretching your hands to many arm, shoulder, neck, or upper back stretches. While both knees are into our chest we can do small circles with our
knees.

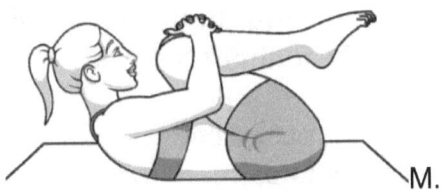

M.

Next, we can do gentle windshield wiper movements with our feet on the bed, with our arms straight out our sides for support, allowing our knees to slowly fall from one side to the other while keeping our back flat on the mattress(Image N). Our tailbone should be tucked under in a neutral position, with our core engaged.

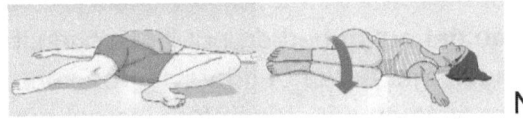

N.

Remember to use smaller movements when we are first waking or getting up. If there is soreness or pain only bring the knees into the chest, and if you feel okay, do small circles with your knees. Do this for a couple of days before attempting to add any twisting motions. We should not do twisting movements when we are in pain. Our intelligent body is the ultimate doctor and will use discomfort and even pain to tell us exactly what it does and does not want us to do. This communication, discomfort and pain, aka symptoms, guides us to better meet the needs of our body. This information in this book is a good starting point, but your body may require slight variations and special requirements to meet its' specific needs. Consult with us or your chosen health professional to help you determine your body's' specific needs.

It is important, with any stretch or activity we perform that we warm up and start with smaller movements first because we always want to be warmed up before we go into deeper movements and stretches. If we have different activities we enjoy doing, like fishing, bowling…, don't wait for the season, train your body to perform those activities throughout the year.

As we turn to our side to get out of bed we can do a little side stretch by using the back of our elbow or forearm(for more of a stretch) to hold the side of our upper body away from the bed, as the side of our hip and leg rest on the bed. Then move to the foot of the bed to stretch the other side(Image O).

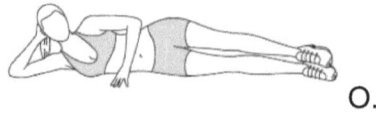

O.

When you are ready to get out of bed do not kick yourself up if you are lying on your back. You should get out of bed by lying on your side first. It is also important when we are lying on our side before we get out of bed to not push with the elbow we are lying on and use our shoulder muscles. The body is too heavy to be lifted by our shoulder alone and this could cause a shoulder injury. Either side we sleep on is fine, but some people may have an injury that needs to be taken into account. The best way to get out of bed is by lying on our side and allowing our feet to come off the bed while the hand from the top arm pushes off the bed. This will cause our body to teeter on our bottom to a sitting position without having to use our shoulder, stomach, or back(Image P).

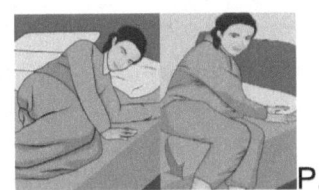
P.

Once sitting we should take a couple of seconds to sit up tall, engage the core and go through mild gentle range of motion exercises with our neck and back to pump the discs and get them ready for gravity(Image Q).

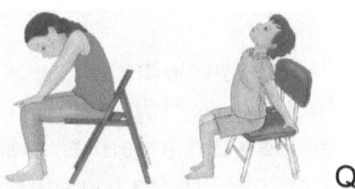
Q.

Now it's time to get up, with our head and shoulders over our hips and our hips over our feet we can stand using our legs. We can also use our hands to push off the top of our legs to keep weight off our back. We want to use our legs as much as possible and our back as little as possible. Getting up from bed can be another winning moment in the quest for the 24-hour workout.

There are 3 ranges of motion our neck (cervical and upper thoracic spine) and back (mid-lower thoracic and lumbar spine) need to be stretched in each and every day. They are flexion(neck:head down/back:bend forward at the waist) and extension(neck:head

back/back:body reaching tall), right(neck:tilt right ear towards right shoulder/back:tilt upper body towards right hip) and left(neck:tilt left ear towards left shoulder/back:tilt upper body towards left hip) lateral flexion, and right(neck:turn face towards the right/back:turn chest towards the right) and left(neck:turn face towards the left/back:turn chest towards the left) rotation.

GETTING READY FOR THE DAY

OK, let's get this day started! Before we went to bed we took a couple minutes to release stress, which allowed us to have a better night's sleep, and we took a couple minutes to warm up in the morning, so we already have 8 great hours of winning moments. These winning moments are reducing stress and promoting better health before we even get out of bed. It is very important to note that this is an ongoing process. We are not looking for perfection, just progress. We will have good days and bad days, and today is a great day to start again. We do not have to win every moment for our health to improve. It's all about winning more moments consistently over a lifetime.

We begin to lose the health benefits we received from exercise, therapy's, and nutrition the day we stop doing those healthy habits. The good news is that the day we start a healthy habit is the day we begin to plant and in time harvest health benefits from those habits.

We can suffer less, experience better health, have more energy, and enjoy a more active life, by winning moments in our day. If we can see our daily activities in this way and apply these principles, anything is possible. Good habits are a lifetime journey and once you experience the health benefits, you will begin to see the impact these moments have on your health and life. Winning moments for better health does not require any additional time from your schedule, it actually adds time. The power of winning moments comes from repurposing the same activities that cause you problems and takes energy from your day, into moments that now lead to more energy and better health in every area of your life.

Having a consistent awareness for winning moments is a process that leads to a healthy lifestyle. The more reminders and visual cues we utilize to improve our awareness the better.

Let's head to the bathroom to brush our teeth, wash our face, put on makeup, brush hair, shave... Don't keep the toothbrush, toothpaste, face towel, makeup, hairbrush, razor etc, in a place that causes you to lean over, bend, or twist. Put these items in a place that is easy to reach while standing in a power posture with the core slightly engaged(Image R). Our body is not warmed up enough to lean over, bend, or twist. These type of motions can irritate the spine. If we need to lean over the sink, make sure there is a place to put one foot up on a low stool or under the sink. If you can't put one leg up, bend both legs and squat down(Image S), don't keep your legs straight and bend over while using your back muscles.

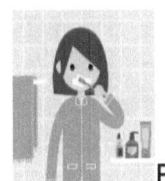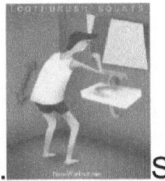

R. S.

When we have both legs straight and we are leaning forward with all our weight on the low back we are in a very vulnerable position for injury. Our legs should always be doing the work while focusing on keeping our back in a power posture and engaged. If you want to add balance work to brushing your teeth in the morning or evening stand up tall with a power posture, engage the core, and balance on one foot, keep the leg you are standing on slightly bent(Image T). This will create core strength, balance, improve brain health, and add some fun. Balance is an important part of health and something we can all work on throughout our day. Standing in line is also a great place to work on balance and win moments.

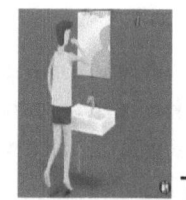

T.

We want to try and do everything we possibly can in a power posture by keeping our head over our shoulders, shoulders over our hips, and hips over our legs, with our legs slightly bent(you do not want to lock your legs), and the core engaged.

I am not a big fan of bathroom talk, but I have heard enough people mention getting in trouble either getting on or off the toilet or somewhere in between, so I'm willing to go there with you. The best way to start is by standing over the toilet, with your feet a little wider apart, straddling the toilet if you need to, so you are in a position to squat straight down. Gently sit on the seat with your back up straight(Image U). When your feet are wider or you are straddling the toilet, your legs are much stronger and you will have better balance, making it a great way to stand up from the toilet as well.

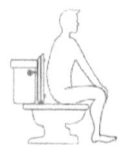

U.

We want to minimize leaning the upper body forward while reaching our bottom back for the seat. Also, we don't want to be far away from the toilet because if we go to far back on our heels we may slam down on the seat.

The proper way to sit and get up from the toilet is feet wider, back up tall, with a power posture and the core slightly engaged.

This is not only a winning moment to build strength and a power posture, but you'll notice your ability to eliminate will improve. When getting up from the toilet seat, with our feet wide, we want to move our bottom forward on the seat the best we can so we can stand up using our legs. If we need to use our arms, it is better to have supports at our sides so our weight stays over our legs. Another option is to push on the tops of our legs with our hands for added support. Be careful not to stretch too far forward to lean on or pull on a counter, this puts weight on our back and can be dangerous. When standing and going number one, stand as close as possible to the toilet. This will allow you to stand up straighter without missing your mark. The last thing anyone wants to do is be too far away from the toilet, one because nobody wants to have to clean it, but two because we don't want to put unnecessary stress on the back or nerves, like the sciatic nerve, by having to lean back too far to reach the toilet or urinal.

Chapter 2

HOURS 10-12

SPIRITUAL, MENTAL, AND PHYSICAL TRAINING/GETTING IN THE SHOWER OR TUB/ DESIGN YOUR HOME FOR HEALTH/ GETTING DRESSED/ SHOES/ ORTHOTICS/ WALLETS/ POCKETBOOKS/BACKPACKS/HOW TO SIT/OPENING DOORS/ GETTING IN-OUT OF CAR/SITTING IN THE CAR/LONG DRIVES/CHIROPRACTIC ADJUSTMENTS

SPIRITUAL, MENTAL, AND PHYSICAL TRAINING

Every winning moment leads to better spiritual, mental, and physical health.

This is the most important time in my day, it's a time we can invest in ourselves spiritually, mentally, and physically. It's the most important and powerful time of the day because it makes every aspect of our day better. This is the time of day that I like to read my *bible*, books, drink my first glass of water, get my chiropractic adjustment, do my breathing, exercise, and have a green's drink. Workouts can vary from day to day and person to person. *The focus and foundation of all my workouts are the health of my spine and discs, the health of my brain and nervous system, and the flexibility, strength, balance, and endurance of my muscular system, which includes my heart.* A power posture, strong core, and flexibility are the best place for everyone to start. Posture, spine health, and flexibility, including chiropractic adjustments and soft tissue work, are some of the most important keys to better health. Unfortunately, they can also be the most overlooked and left out aspects of many peoples exercise programs. A Power Posture is looking at ourselves in a mirror so that from the front view of ourselves, the middle of our forehead, nose, and chin line up straight down the middle of our chest, and straight down between the middle of our legs. When visualizing a power poster from the side, our ear should be over the middle of our shoulder, and our shoulder over the middle of our hips, our hips should be over our knees, and our ankles. Many people use the term core and core engagement. It is important that we understand what core means and how to maximize the strength, flexibility, endurance, and balance of our core. The center of our core is around the belly button area. It begins with, the pudendal muscle, the muscle between your legs that you contract to stop going to the bathroom or for kegel exercises, up to where your muscles attach to your ribcage, which is right below your chest. These muscles go all the way around our body including the front, sides, and back of our body. Some of the muscles or on the surface and some are deep in our body. The way to create a power posture is by being in the proper posture, while gently engaging all the muscles of the core. I even like to extend the core to be my posture all the way out the top of my head, my arms and legs, to out the bottom of my feet. This is more of a mental exercise to ensure that every body part is supporting a power posture and engaged, ready for work and to handle good(exercise) or bad stress.

We want all our core muscles to have balance, flexibility, strength, and endurance. When working on the core think of an X. The core muscles that make the X are our abdominal muscles and gluteal muscles/hamstrings make one line of the X, and the other line of the X is made of the low back muscles and our hip flexors/quadriceps. If you look at these muscles in an anatomy book you will see how the middle of the X, where the lines cross, would be right in the center of our core(Image V). All these muscles need to be addressed if we want to have a strong core.

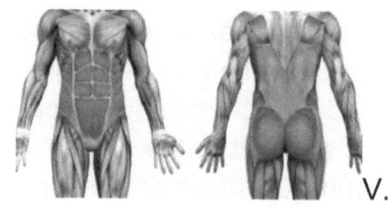

V.

My favorite core workout is in a pool. I can work my entire core while maintaining a power posture. When swimming, using the kickboard, or using flippers while kicking on my belly or back helps me build strength, flexibility, endurance, and balance in my core that would be hard to recreate on land. Gravity, or working out on land, usually causes you to work some muscle more than others, causing you to have to do multiple exercises to get all the muscles of the core. In the pool, you can make slight variations and give more attention to any muscle group in your core that you want. In the water you can work your core longer and with less rest, keeping more tension on the muscles for longer periods of time. The large amount of stimulation to the hips from kicking is great because it stimulates the nerve system to help solidify the posture I am working out in.

My workouts include walking, hiking, biking, water workouts, swimming, surfing, stretching, breathing, different styles of yoga(I use Sean Vigue Fitness on Youtube for yoga, pilates, stretching, alignment, balance, and body weight exercises...Thanks Sean), balance work, weight training, rubber bands, core work, wobble chair, trigger stick, foam roller, inversion table, combinations of all the above, chiropractic adjustments... Basically, anything that gets me moving and promotes growth, health, and a positive attitude. Like I mentioned, I do enjoy working out in water, it is a great form of resistance that stays consistent throughout the entire range of motion of the exercise. The water is where I do most of my back, shoulders, arms, and core work. I also do chest and leg workouts too. While exercising in the water it also allows you to maintain a neutral position and power posture at all times, while protecting the muscle you are not using. You can do stretches on the side of the pool and gentle stretches as you move your arms through the water. I have hand paddles I can use to add resistance or use to twist and strengthen rotation of my core. I can also use the water to do muscles scans, while exercising, to see where there is tightness, resistance, or soreness, so I know where to focus with my adjustments, posture work, stretching, and soft tissue work. When I find a spot, I work both sides of the body to restore balance. Working out in the water started for me when I was living in pain each day. I could not walk, sit, or even lay down without pain. In the pool, I would do light walking in place, my upper body workouts, and I would swim with just my upper body because it was too painful to kick. That was 20 years ago. The pool really helped me to stay active when I was suffering and is one of the many things I still enjoy to this day.

This is what my goals are for a week:
Most Days to Everyday: Bible, Wobble Chair, Spinal Range Of Motion, Cervical Curve Work, Trigger Stick, Foam Roller, Inversion, Deep Breathing, Stretching, Balance Work, Some Form of Exercise, Fruits and Vegetables.
2-3 Days a Week: Focus on Strength and Soft Tissue Work:
Stretching/Balance/Yoga/Pilates/Trigger Stick/Foam Roller, Resistance Training with Bodyweight/Weights/Rubber Bands/Resistance Paddles in Pool, Core Work, Activities: Hiking/Walks, Swimming, Biking, Boogie Boarding, Surfing...the activities are mixed and matched based on the season.
1 Day a Week: Chiropractic Adjustment

On busy days I have to get very creative and find things that fit into the natural flow of that day. A busy day may involve doing a set of push-ups here or there, squats while standing at the computer, lunges while writing at a desk, or a balance pose instead of standing. Core work may need to be done while sitting or working on the computer. I will use a foam roller instead of a chair, a quick trigger stick session as a 30 second break, and if possible, get on the inversion table while answering emails and texts. Stretches while reading...something, anything, whenever possible, even if it takes the whole day to get a couple sets completed. If I am really pressed for time I will get a chiropractic adjustment because they can reduce the most stress in the shortest amount of time by keeping the pathway clear from the brain to the body. However, my best days are the days when I make the time, even if I have to get up earlier than I would like, to make sure I spend time in the Bible and investing in my health.

This is the proper time and place to safely work on posture, spine health, strength, flexibility, endurance, and balance for all our muscle groups.

A big focus of my training in the quest for the 24-hour workout is to maintain a power posture when I exercise and prepare my body to be stronger, more flexible, and better prepared for anything that can happen on any given day. We even need to be prepared as much as possible for any surprises. We know that on any day surprises can happen like stepping off the curb wrong, having to reach further for a coat than expected in the back seat of a car, picking up a water jug, and the list goes on. If we know surprises happen each day, it makes sense that we prepare our body the best we can.

Spiritual, Mental, and Physical training may have nothing to do with what we do, but has everything to do with how well we do it.

GETTING IN THE SHOWER OR TUB
When getting in the shower or tub take small steps getting in and out, do not overstretch or over rotate the back, hips, or knees. Make sure the floor and tub or shower surface is not slippery. If it is you may want to consider getting a non-slip surface, like a shower mat. While showering put one foot up at a time to wash each leg or shave. If you drop anything make sure to bend with your knees to pick it up, try not to lean over using only your back. Use your legs to stand up and be careful not to hit a soap dish, nozzle, or facet on the way down or up. Some people like to do lite stretching as the warm water hits their muscles.

DESIGN YOUR HOME FOR HEALTH

It's a great idea to set up our bedroom, bathroom, kitchen, living room, den, office, garage and shed so our most used items or heavier items that we may need to lift are in the drawers, racks, shelves, or hung at the height of our chest or midsection. Keep the least used items in the lower or higher spaces and places. Be very careful not to bend over, pull on a drawer and twist all at the same time. Compound movements, two or more movements together, like bending, leaning, and twisting put a lot of stress on the spine, discs, and muscles. When we add pulling to a compound movement (multiple movements at one time) we increase our risk for unnecessary stress and possible injury to the back. I mention all that to say, squat down in front of lower drawers or bend down onto one knee and pull drawers evenly.

Preparing every environment for better health makes being healthy easier.

GETTING DRESSED

They say "you're never fully dressed without a smile", but if you are living in pain it can be hard to smile. *The same way we get dressed to avoid pain is the same way we get dressed to stay healthy, a power posture with core engagement.* So here are some tips to help with getting dressed. Picking clothes can really help you heal faster if you are suffering and in pain, and that's a big win. Looser clothes are easier to get off and on and comfortable slip-on shoes can help avoid bending. Always make sure sleeves and pant legs are untangled before they are put on. If you have neck or shoulder problems, looser tops that button or zip will be less stress on the neck and shoulders. When choosing pants, it's about the pant legs. The easier you can get your foot out the bottom of the pant leg, and less resistance there is pulling the pants up the better. If you are really struggling to put on your socks or pants, because of pain, you can put them on while lying on your back. Another option is to put your socks and pants on while sitting. You can pull one knee at a time into your chest putting your heel up on the edge of the bed, this will also give you a nice stretch. The goal would be to get your foot fully in your sock and then work your foot out the bottom of the pant leg before you put your foot down gently. If you like to lean forward while sitting on the edge of the bed to put socks or pants on, when you're ready to get up, put both hands on the top of your legs and push with your hands so that your back isn't the only thing lifting the upper body to a sitting position. A good stretch when putting on socks is while sitting, place the outside of the ankle of the leg your lifting, on top of the other leg that is bent with the foot on the floor. When you are done putting your sock on, lean forward for a nice stretch which is great for many people with low back, hip, and sciatica pain(Image W). Remember to always stretch both sides and to use your hands to press back up from stretching to the sitting position.

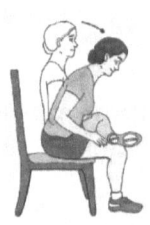

W.

A person's ability to do things they were not able to do before, like putting on their socks, is a good sign of improvement.

It is important to find a way to get dressed that causes the least amount of stress to our body. Sometimes it's first dressing the arm or leg that hurts the most, sometimes it's dressing it last. Sometimes it's getting both arms or legs in position, with the clothing just a little on each arm or leg, then working the clothing on. Other times it's getting one arm or leg all the way into the piece of clothing before the other. The main point is that we learn from our body's by experimenting to determine the best way to get dressed with the least amount of irritation. When it comes to getting dressed we want to be in a position that causes the least amount of stress, however, we want to make sure we are stable and secure. This is important because we don't want to find ourselves balancing on one foot, in pain, when our foot gets stuck in a pant leg, and we end up having to hop on one leg so we don't fall, or worse, we do fall(Image X). If standing feels better, use a dresser for balance and support. Try not to bend down to the point of pain while getting dressed(Image X). If possible we should find something to pull up our pants, like a hanger. The key to putting on pants is to make sure our foot is all the way out of the bottom of the pant leg before we make our move. Sudden and unexpected movements, like fighting with a foot that is standing on a pant leg can cause pain.

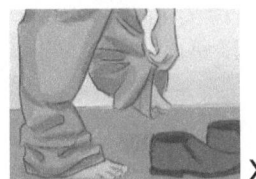

X.

When putting on our shoes it is all about how we took them off the last time we wore them. When we take off our shoes make sure that we put our foot on a chair or stair, make the laces very loose so we can slip our feet out of the shoes when we put them both safely back on the ground. The next time we put our shoes on we will be able to slip them on. Then, bring one foot at a time up onto a chair or stair to tie each shoe(Image Y).

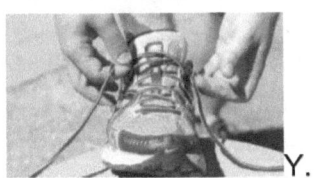

Y.

If we didn't take off our shoes that way, somehow we or someone else can loosen the laces so we can slip our feet into the shoes and tie them on a chair or stair. One good way to loosen our laces is to bend down on one knee utilizing a chair or support as we bend down and get back up. The support should be used on the same side as the knee we are bending down on. If we are close enough to the support and it is stable(!!) we can lean against it to take some weight off our body. Once balanced, loosen the other shoelace. Switch sides to do the other shoe. If we are on the right knee, the support should be on the right, to loosen left shoe. If we are on the left knee, the support should be on the left, to loosen right shoe(Image Z).

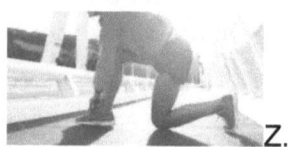

Z.

SHOES

I can not stress enough the importance of shoes. *Shoes determine how our body handles every impact and interaction with the ground and how that stress enters our body.* These stresses have an effect on our feet, ankles, knees, legs, hips, back, neck, head...everything. I had some shoes that reminded me that I have a back and caused back pain, which I try to never wear again. However, I have one brand of shoe that allows me to enjoy the great outdoors, take walks, workout, stand all day at work, run errands, without feeling any stress on my back. These are the only style of shoes I ever wear no matter the weather, the situation, or the dress code. My back, feeling good, and being active is a priority to me, so my shoes are not negotiable. I am not necessarily promoting a brand, however, I am promoting the lifestyle that my shoes provide for me. I found them by not wearing shoes that bothered my back until I found shoes that didn't. I noticed I would wear these shoes for different activities for longer and longer periods of time and still feel good. Once I found them, I kept buying them, because they work for me. It is important to listen to your body so you can find the shoes that work for you. Look at different shoes and try them based off shoes that you have liked the most in the past. If you have never found shoes you like, then try different shoes until you find ones you really like. Try shoes with a heel(like a running shoe), try without a heel(like a hiking shoe), try soft, try firm, try different arch supports, try different widths, try different brands. You will know when you find the right shoe, they make a noticeable difference by reducing stress on your body while allowing you to be more active.

ORTHOTICS

Orthotics and heel lifts are another great gift to your feet and body, they are inserts that you put in your shoes. *These are specific for your feet and body type and take into consideration the arch of your feet, alignment of your feet, ankles, knees, hips, spine, shoulders, neck, and head.* You should get a proper analysis of your feet, including a scan of your feet and an x-ray analysis of your spine and hip heights to find the best pair for you. They are great for your feet, ankles, knees, and hips, but they also take a lot of pressure off your spine and promote better posture by creating better alignment when you stand and with every step you take.

When we have pain or even if we do not, it is always better to wear good shoes.

WALLETS/POCKETBOOKS/BACKPACKS
The easiest rule to follow is the thinner the wallet and the lighter the pocketbook or backpack the better. Never keep a wallet in your back pocket. It causes your hips and back to get out of alignment causing more stress on your spine, discs, and muscles. The best pocketbooks, for your back, are the ones that are like a backpack or the type that have a long enough strap to go over your head, while the bag stays close to the side of your body, at the height of your core. The closer the pocketbook is to your body the safer it is for your body. Be careful putting the pocketbook on if you have neck or shoulder issue. If you are going to wear your pocketbook on one shoulder, keep the bag close to you, under your arm. You can even hold it like a package so it doesn't pull on your shoulder or cause you neck stress from having to raise that shoulder up trying to make sure the bag doesn't fall off your shoulder. When picking a backpack for a child, the backpack should not be wider or longer than the child's torso. The bag should never go 4 inches below their waist when they are wearing it. The weight of a child's backpack should not be more than 5-10% of their weight. When packing the backpack, heavier items should be closer to the back. Make sure the straps are loose when putting the backpack on so they don't put any unnecessary stress on the shoulders. Always use both straps, a chest strap to secure the two shoulder straps, to hold the backpack on, and a hip strap. While putting on

the backpack, have the child stand up tall and engage their core. Tighten the shoulder straps evenly, so the backpack is close to the body and the weight is distributed evenly in the center of the back, in the upper to mid back area(Image AA).

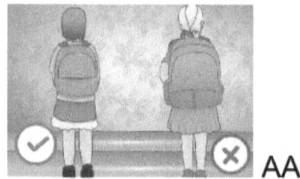 AA.

Be careful with bookbags on rollers, kids can tend to over pack them. They cause kids to twist to one side as they pull these bags and the bag can pull back on them as they get stuck navigating them through obstacles. The rolling bags are also more stress on the shoulder as well, sometimes these bags even roll over twisting the entire arm.

HOW TO SIT
A lot of times I will stand and avoid sitting whenever possible, however, if we're are going to sit, one suggestion would be to try a balance ball. With the balance ball, our core will stay engaged, our brain will be firing, and if we keep a power posture we'll be getting stronger and healthier as we sit, winning more moments. *If we're going to use a chair*, we want to position our back as far back into the chair as possible, bringing our legs around the side of the chair, like sitting on a horse. Sit up tall and allow the back of the chair to be a guide, but we still need to use our core muscles to strengthen our posture. If the chair is too deep to reach the back, sit on the front edge of the chair, sit up tall while contracting your core and holding a power posture(Image BB). If we are using any type of table (dinner table, coffee table, tv tray) we want to be as close as possible so that we are not leaning over to reach the table or losing our posture as we sit. There are many great stretches to counteract the negative effects of sitting. They are stretches that focus on the stomach and hip flexors, including the psoas muscle. If you want a great stretch, do a lunge on both sides of your body for 30 seconds

after you have been sitting. If you have a foam roller or trigger stick you can roll out your thighs, hip flexors, and stomach.

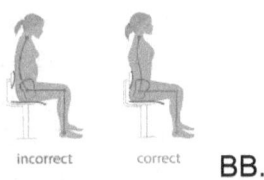

incorrect   correct   BB.

Always leave a little more time than needed for traveling to work, the gym, or chiropractic adjustment. Giving ourselves extra time to travel places will always produce better health and more enjoyment than rushing, stress, and worry.

OPENING DOORS

I know when I leave the house I can have so many things in my hands that I am trying to open the door with anything other than my hands. Then I use my elbow to pry the door open, my foot to kick the screen door open, then I have to do a fast spin so the screen door doesn't come back and hit my elbow, but instead, it hits my back. There are other times where we pull on doors that are heavy or stuck as we go in and out of our homes or any of the other different doors we go through in a day. So here it is, the right way to open doors for better health. *I think of opening doors, like doing a one arm row at a gym.* If the door handle is on the left, I have my left leg in front of my body and to the left of the door. My right foot is behind my body, with the front of my right leg practically in line with the door handle. I am standing as close to the door as possible, but so it can still open. I stand up as straight as I can and place my right hand on the handle and my left hand safely on the door frame. In a power posture, I engage my core, shoulders, and arms and pull with my legs and arm straight back. I try not to twist my back or use my shoulders more than necessary. If the handle is on the right, I reverse my positioning to open the door the same way. If it is a sliding door position yourself to slide the door towards your body.

GETTING IN-OUT OF CAR, SITTING IN THE CAR, AND LONG DRIVES
Getting in the car by putting one leg in at a time can cause a lot of stress on your back, hips, and knees. *First, sit down in the car, before bringing your legs into the car.* You can use your hands as support on the seat as you lower yourself into the car, watch your head! At this point, both feet should be out in front of you, outside of the car. Make sure the door is close so you don't have to reach as far once you are in the car. Now, little by little rotate on your bottom on the car seat until both feet are in the car. Engage the core and shoulder as you lean over to shut the car door.

Car seats have a number of adjustments on them. *Start by sitting up tall and being supported by the chair, but stay in a power posture keeping the core engaged.* We don't want to be too relaxed and have the chair do all the work. One reason is to protect our back so that any bumps in the road go into the muscles instead of our spine. Driving is also another opportunity to strengthen the core and solidify our power posture. Sitting close to the steering wheel allows us to keep our posture, without having to reach forward, round our shoulders, and stretch our neck and back forward to reach the wheel or pedals. While driving we can either contract and relax the core or contract and hold the core for sets. We can also do abdominal or ab work, low back work, and spinal disc hydration. While exhaling tuck the tail (think of the bones we sit on) under while contracting the belly button back towards the spine. Then on the inhale push the tail back to a neutral position, contract the core while lifting up the midsection, and pushing the chest forward. Do not arch the back too much, it is more about sitting tall than about leaning backward. Always use your abdominals and the muscles on the sides of your core to protect your back. This creates a pumping motion in the low back that helps the spine and discs while also working the abs and low back. It is also good on longer drives to change the seat position so that we use different muscles in different ways during our drive time. When getting out of the car, hold onto the door and keep it close, so the wind doesn't catch it and cause you to reach or get pulled by the car door. Bring both feet out of the car, before you stand up. Once both feet are out of the car, move closer towards the edge of the side of the seat and stand up over your feet. A great stretch to counteract the stress of driving and sitting is a psoas or lunge type of stretch(Image CC(start slow and over time add the back leg lift for a deeper stretch)). Keep your head and chest up as you stretch forward. Never let your knee get in front of your ankle on the front leg, square your hips forward, while getting into a gentle stretch. Imagine your breath going into the muscle on your inhale and on your exhale, relaxing the muscle, letting your breath guide the stretch. Always do both sides when you stretch. *The number one key to long drives is to get out of the car and walk a little bit as often as possible.*

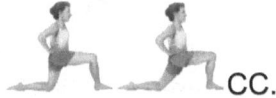

CC.

It's not how long you walk when we get up from sitting, it's how often we get up from sitting to walk that offers the greatest health benefits. This is true for any type of sitting, whether it be on a couch, chair, at a desk, or in a car.

If you have time, once you get to where you are going, park in a location that allows for a nice walk. It doesn't have to be long, just enough to get the blood and joints of your body pumping, and time to clear your mind, so you can have a positive mindset and impact on your daily activities and in the lives of others.

Moving the joints of our body is one of the fastest ways to promote a positive attitude and perspective.

CHIROPRACTIC ADJUSTMENTS

Every area of our health requires attention and care. Heart, lungs, muscles, skin, hair, teeth, neck, back, arm, legs, everything. If we stop caring for any part of our body that is the day the health of that body part will begin to prematurely decline. The one reason our spine needs to be at the top of our list of body parts to take care of is that it determines how well our brain is able to meet the needs of our body and the body's' ability to communicate those needs to the brain. The needs of every cell! The cells that fight cancer, get nutrition from foods, tell the heart to beat, and the lungs to breath, every single function our body performs each and every second of each and every day. The impulses or life that transmit through the brain and nerves travel through and are protected by the spine. A healthy spine and power posture means a clear path for those impulses and healthy communication that results in maximum power being expressed in each cell. This is the same power that made the body, performs all the functions in the body, and heals and repairs the body. An unhealthy spine or posture, a subluxated spine, clogs the path for brain and nerve impulses to the body and those impulses from the body to the brain. These subluxations weaken impulses causing the development of weaker cells, tissues, organs, organ systems, and over time leading to a weaker body. This weaker body will be more susceptible to injury, slower to recover, less able to fight disease, making it difficult to properly perform normal functions, making it impossible for a person to enjoy their best life. Over time this can lead to dysfunction and dis-ease. The spine needs to be cared for each day with proper posture, stretches, range of motion exercises and strengthening. However, unhealthy spinal joints, subluxated joints, can be irritated by the same movements we use to keep spinal joints healthy. *The chiropractor can find unhealthy spinal joints and postures, called subluxations, and provide a chiropractic adjustment to those areas allowing them, over time, to become healthy again.* Most importantly these chiropractic adjustments clear the path between the brain and body which are vital and the foundation of all health. The ultimate goal, once the spine is adjusted and healthy, is to be checked for subluxations once or twice a month depending on your body's needs to help those joints in your spine that are not moving like the others or have gotten stuck. This can happen in many different ways throughout your day. Spinal subluxations are caused by mental, physical, and chemical stresses. I see many people that say I don't know what happened or why I am in pain, I didn't do anything out of the ordinary. When you get chiropractic adjustments regularly and unlock the spine from new injuries or subluxations, even mico injuries, you get the added benefit of not allowing that injury to remain in your spine an extended period of time, which would mean anything over 2 weeks. Injuries that remain in the spine for 2 weeks or more begin to cause arthritis of the spine, disc disease, and irritation or weakening to the nerve system.

There are 3 basic levels of improvement a person will experience when they begin to receive chiropractic adjustments. Some go through these levels faster, some slower, some people even skip levels. Level 1 is relief which can happen on the first adjustment, but it is safer to say most people will see a noticeable change within two weeks. Remember some people, even if their pain just started, are coming in with years of spine and disc degeneration. Level 2 is consistent relief, when people are starting to have more good days, than bad. This is when people are getting back to their lives, however, they can feel so much better that they may aggravate their problem by trying to get back to full speed to fast. An encouraging sign of level 2 is when episodes of discomfort or pain are less intense, less often, and any episodes of discomfort or pain goes away faster, while the person is able to be more active. Level 3 is when the person is not only healthier than they were before the injury, but their health continues to improve as they begin doing things they stopped doing years ago because of discomfort or pain. Level 3 is where people begin to realize they are living a better life with chiropractic care.

These chiropractic adjustments allow us to get the most out of each and every spinal joint, which in turn, allows us to get the most from the impulses for health that travel from our brain, through our spine, and to our body. This means that chiropractic adjustments allow us to experience better health. They also help to ensure we get more out of the spinal exercises we are performing each day.

Chapter 3

HOURS 12-21

DESIGN YOUR WORKPLACE FOR HEALTH/STAY AT HOME PARENT/COMPUTER/DESK/WORKING WITH YOUR HANDS/ON YOUR FEET A LOT/LIFT/SHOVEL/VACUUM/SWEEP/THE LITTLE THINGS/POWER LUNCH/BREAK/FREETIME

DESIGN YOUR WORKPLACE FOR HEALTH

Let's look at our workplace and the activities that we have to do as if we were looking at different equipment in the gym. Any opportunity we have to improve posture, engage the core, strengthen a muscle, or safely perform a stretch, we should do it!

Due to the amount of time you spend at work, minimal effort in this area with consistency will show maximum results.

Many jobs have similar stresses on the body, so the fundamentals for winning moments at work can apply to many different jobs or areas of life. One good thing about applying the concept of exercise to any daily activity or kind of work is that it has been proven that one way muscles are strengthened is based on the time the muscle is under tension. The work environment is a great opportunity to exercise your muscles in proper positions and power postures for long periods of time. Don't miss this opportunity for better health.

STAY AT HOME PARENT

This is one of the areas that you can be very creative based on the age of your children. *I would do squats, lunges, and burpees pushing my daughter on the swing. If you like to run you can play tag. I have had many different jungle gym workouts. If you are waiting during your child's class or game you can do some deep breathing, stretching, find an activity to do like push-ups, wall sits or balancing on one foot.* Don't worry about how it will look, make health more important. It would be a shame to waste 20 or 30 minutes or more of your time, when you can enjoy some exercise, recharge, and encourage others. Important Point: I do know how important eye contact is with our children to acknowledge our love and support for their efforts and growth, they love knowing we see them, so we need to make it a top priority that we are available, even if it is while doing some breathing, stretching, wall sits or squats. Most importantly this is a powerful time to teach our children how to be healthy. They need to learn how to, in a fun way, win moments that lead to a better healthier, more active life. We can stretch with them, walk and talk, make action movies, play outdoors with other families as a family, make a game out of yard work, or other projects that need to be done.

Schedule active lunches with friends before drop off and pick up. If you have a good friend divide and conquer things you both need to do to save time, so you have more time. We don't always need to compartmentalize our lives, we can turn things we need to do into an exercise, like doing the laundry or picking up toys. More than anything else our family wants our time and attention, so our only job is to make what needs to get done enjoyable. If you need a gift, turn it into an art project with the kids, where you go on a hike to find items, then make a gift they'll never forget from those items. Creativity is a great brain exercise.

Look for ways to win at the game of life.

COMPUTER/DESK (Work or Home)

If you work on a computer or at a desk set up your workstation to promote a power posture. *Your head should be over your shoulders, with your body close to the desk to avoid reaching. Keep your knees and hips bent at 90 degrees, with the computer screen lifted so you are able to look right in front of you at eye level to see the entire screen, without having to look down. You can move the keyboard, up or down, in or out, to accommodate good posture.* Everything you need should be right in front of you so that you do not have to turn or twist for long periods of time. *Your elbows should have a nice natural bend around 90 degrees as well. Your forearms should be in a straight line with your wrists and hands when you are typing or using a mouse*(Image DD).

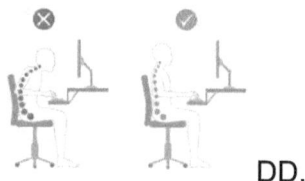

DD.

Throughout the day stretch your neck, shoulders, arms, wrists, hands, and back to stop stress from building up and to promote health. Many people are also using standing workstations(Image EE) or sitting on an exercise ball while they work at their desk.

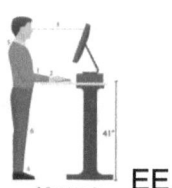

EE.

WORKING WITH YOUR HANDS

If you work a lot with your hands, which includes, computer work, using a mouse, phone, pad, sewing, needlepoint, gripping things like hammers, screwdrivers, or other tools, writing, anything that requires you to use your hands, this is for you. These type of activities, day after day, can cause finger, hand, wrist, forearm, elbow, arm, shoulder, and even neck pain and headaches. It is important that we care for our hands, wrists, and forearms like any other part of our body. *Because many of our hand problems come from gripping, closing our hands, it helps to do exercises and stretches that balance those muscles by doing things that open our hands.* A rubber band is an easy way to help balance our forearms, wrists, and hands by lengthening the tight muscles and strengthening the overstretched ones. With your hand in the shape of a claw, put the rubber band around the outside of your fingers, right above the base of your fingernails. Open and close the claw. You should feel the tension on the top of the forearm if you are doing it correctly. This will help counteract the stresses of all the things we do gripping and closing our hands and can help with many things including carpal tunnel type symptoms. It also helps to do stretches and massage to balance out all the muscles of your hands, wrists, and forearms. Foam roller, trigger stick, golf ball, frozen water bottle, any instrument that can help relieve tight and tender spots or to keep your hands, wrist, and forearms healthy are good. You can roll or press them on your hands and forearms, if you find any areas of discomfort, spend some extra time in that area. I use the trigger stick to roll over my forearms and wrists as often as possible. Of course don't forget to care for your neck, shoulders, and arms if you are working with your hands a lot.

Cell phone use can cause a lot of stress on a person's neck, hands, wrists, and especially thumbs with swiping. Do your best to take care of these areas, work both sides equally, and rest them regularly, especially when they are irritated.

ON YOUR FEET A LOT

The feet and calves need love too. They do a lot of work in a day. *Stretches for your calves and feet will make a difference, so I will share a couple I do.* The calves need to be stretched in both directions. It is important that you start slow, with stretching your foot and calf, by putting the ball of your foot on a step and letting your heal gently lower down. Remember to do both sides, but also to stretch the front of your feet and calves. You can achieve this when you point your toes and foot down and you feel a stretch on the front of your legs and feet. You can use the ground to add a little more to the stretch, by putting the top of your toes on the ground and stretching your foot forward.   After some time, for a deeper stretch, while on your knees you can sit on your feet. Sit on your heels with the top of the foot on the ground to stretch the front of your feet and calves and sit on your heels with the toes and balls of your feet on the ground to stretch the bottom of your feet and back of your calves. Stretching and massage are also good for your feet and calves too. Foam roller, trigger stick, golf ball, frozen water bottle, any instrument that can help relieve tight and tender spots or to keep feet and calves healthy are good. You can roll or press them on your feet and calves, if you find any areas of discomfort, spend some extra time in that area. I have a foam roller with knobs on it, so after I do my calves, I stand and roll one foot on it at a time, to work on the bottom of my feet. Of course don't forget to care for your back, legs, hips, and core if you are on your feet all day.

LIFT/SHOVEL/VACUUM/SWEEP (Work or Home)

When lifting at home or work remember to warm up and stretch. Try not to lift or do more than you are used to doing, especially if your body has not had to do that activity before or in a while. There is a chance it may not be prepared for that activity and vulnerable to injury, so warming up and stretching first is vital. It is also important to take care of ourselves on a regular basis prior to any activity, this way if we ask our body to do more than usual we are better prepared. I do understand how life works and that it is not that simple, but I wanted to give you something to think about. It is important that we do our part to avoid injury or better prepare our body for all the unknowns in life that happen each day.

So, here is how we should *lift, shovel, vacuum, sweep...any activity that requires the use of our entire body* at one time.
Once you have warmed up and stretched, start with a power posture with the core engaged. All our joints should be slightly bent, but firm and ready for work. That means shoulders, elbows, wrists, hands, fingers, hips, knees, ankles, feet, and toes. Muscles like to be worked, plus it is good for them. Muscles also protect the joints of our body from being overstretched or pulled beyond what is safe for them. It is important that whenever we are performing an activity that we do not fully extend our shoulders, elbows, hips,

knees or any other body part. We want to keep all our joints safe. Also, please don't push boxes our objects on the floor with your foot, it can stress your knee, hip, and/or back. Whenever possible use a hand truck, dolly, or sliders to move objects.

Start in a power posture, Core engaged, Joints slightly bent, ALL Muscles engaged

Now when it comes to lifting, sliding heavy objects, vacuuming, or sweeping we want to engage our body as if the task in front of us is heavier or harder than it actually is. This is not just about our backs, it includes engaging every muscle we will use, like your shoulder for example, as you prepare to pull a trash can. This way we will be prepared and not surprised by the weight of the object when we get started. Get as close as possible to the object you are lifting or moving. We always want to do as much work as possible with our legs. Bend the legs as much as possible when lifting something off the ground or table and move the legs as often as possible when transporting lifted objects, sliding objects, shoveling, vacuuming, or sweeping(Images FF).

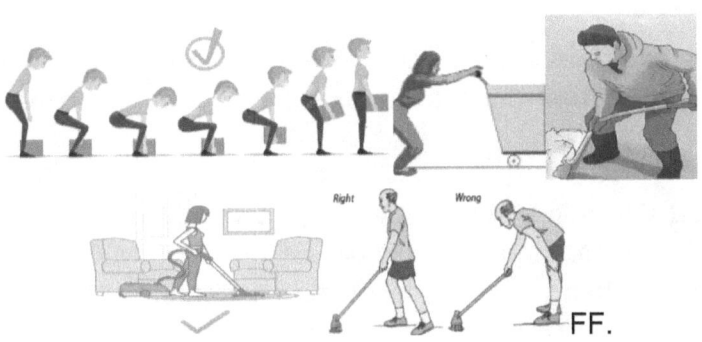

FF.

Perform shorter movements to stay in a posture of power. We should avoid using our upper body whenever possible. When we reach, overextend, tilt, twist...we lose our power posture, the posture that we are the strongest and most protected, and become vulnerable to injury. When putting down an object, place it on a table so you will not have to bend down as far to the ground. This also helps because you will be able to unpack or work with objects from a standing position. If the object needs to be placed on the floor, we want to keep the object close to us and use our legs as much as possible. It is always better to take more trips with lighter weight than to rush to get a job done. If you have a choice, choose to push versus pulling objects that slide across the ground. Get as low as necessary to push the objects so that your hands are somewhere between the level of your chest to above your belly button, depending on the height of the object. If the object isn't moving with pushing, because the front edge is getting stuck on something, never lean over to pull. Stand up in a power position, drop your hips and butt low with your back up tall, with all your muscles engaged, including your core. If the object is light enough, you might want to lift it to a level where you feel stronger and there is less stress on your back. Chart out and clear your path before you start. If two people are lifting an object make sure you are communicating any obstacles like walls, railings, or stairs. Take small steps backward, to stay in a posture of power. Anytime a person loses their power posture, relaxes the core, or makes bigger movements, usually when they are trying to save time or getting tired, that's where most people experience stiffness, tightness, pain, and injury either that day or the next.

It requires less time, less money, and less pain to stay healthy, but it does require more thoughtfulness, discipline, and consistency.

THE LITTLE THINGS
Sneezing and Coughing: *When sneezing or coughing, let the air go out of your body, don't try to stop it or hold any of it in.* Work with your body as you help the air out. When you hold a sneeze or cough in the internal pressure is not good for your body. Let your body move with the sneeze or cough, so less force goes into your body.

POWER LUNCH/BREAK/FREE TIME
Lunchtime, breaks, and free time for me is a time to be active. I like to walk, do push-ups, or stretches. Sometimes I follow a traditional workout, many

times I focus on my trouble areas or tight areas that are revealing themselves throughout the day or areas that may come into play based on the activities I am doing or need to do. I spend time, whenever possible, releasing stress and increasing the flexibility of my muscles so that my body will continue to heal, repair, and work at its' best throughout the entire day. I feel my best lunches, the ones that give me the most energy and focus for the rest of the day, are when I get a chiropractic adjustment, do some soft tissue work, or exercise, even if it's only for 10 minutes. Then after, I like to eat a light healthy lunch. It is a lot easier to eat a healthy lunch after you have released some stress from your morning and your feeling good.

It is a great idea whenever possible to stretch throughout the day.

Chapter 4

HOURS 22-24

FINISH STRONG/RELAX STRONG/SLEEP STRONG/START STRONG/LIVE STRONG

FINISH STRONG

The end of the day is a great time to get everything out of our head and onto paper or a phone so our brain can know that all our important thoughts are in a safe place, which is what it needs to relax. Think of it as a vital brain exercise. Once we organize those thoughts it's time to set them free to our most powerful mind, our unconscious minds, where solutions are waiting. This list we create will be a starting point for tomorrow. An important part of planning is to organize priorities at the top of our list. These are the things that give us what we need to live each day at our highest level. The 2 things I need to do before my family wakes up or day gets started is time with God in the Bible and some form of soft tissue work and/or exercise. There is such a significant difference in everything I do when I start my day this way, that it's beyond explaining. All I can say is prioritizing your list matters! If we move our top priorities down the list, because we are overwhelmed with everything that needs to be done or there isn't enough time for everything, the things that are most important to us can become another box that we have to check. Sometimes half-heartedly, missing out on their power and the reason they are at the top of our list. These priorities are at the top of the list because they make us better and better able to do everything else on our list. Next, we need to plan smart, we don't want to overextend ourselves to do the impossible and it's also important that we remain flexible with our plans. Dream big and start small. The day will provide us every opportunity we need to grow spiritually, mentally, and physically, regardless of if it was or was not on our list. Sometimes the greatest moments that happen in our day are moments that were not on our list. Winning moments include our ability to adapt to any given moment with excellence and our response to unexpected changes to our plans.

A key to winning moments is proper planning along with the ability to be flexible as we manage our schedule and time. A reasonable schedule will create winning moments and an overbooked schedule will complicate them.

When we return home from a long days work the couch or chair may be calling, scratch that, screaming our name. Thinking about doing something else, even something for our health may be the last thing we want to do but could be the difference maker in our journey to better health. These are the types of moments that can change everything. Do you know how many times I've said to myself "aw mannn" as I've had to force myself to invest in my health for 5-10 minutes after a long day? Sometimes just getting started is all I needed and I end up spending 30 minutes, but sometimes it's' barely 5 minutes. However, this is something I am sure of, I have never gotten done and been upset that I took that time. Sometimes you have to go through it before you can look back and see the value, getting started is the hardest part. If we allow any stress from the day to build up while sitting on the couch or chair we will carry those effects into our nights' rest when we go to sleep and even into the next day. These negative effects can compound over time and little by little our health will decline. *However, if we take 5 to 10 minutes before our relaxation time getting a chiropractic adjustment, doing soft tissue work, exercises like sitting on a foam roller or doing a couple stretches, or maybe even taking a little walk around the block, we will get more out of our days efforts, relaxation time, sleep, and a better head start on tomorrow.*

RELAX STRONG
When it is time to relax in your favorite chair or on the couch make sure the tv, laptop, phone, pad, or book is positioned in a way that allows your spine

to be aligned. Also, make sure the chair and couch are being enjoyed in a way that maximizes a power posture and spinal alignment as well.

Proper rest is the best way to start the next day. Clearing our mind, stretching our body, and relaxing is important in our quest for better health.

SLEEP STRONG/START STRONG/LIVE STRONG

Sleeping...The next 6 to 8 hours is body repair, power posture work, and preparing for the activities and day ahead. Getting up in the morning begins the awareness of seeing our day as an opportunity to reach new levels of health with the things that we're already doing, that have always been right in front of us. Our workday offers us the opportunity to turn our body into a fat burning machine while building strength, flexibility, endurance, and balance. Lunch is an opportunity to recharge, get the blood flowing, and release any tight spots. The only thing that's left is to finish the day strong. Winning moments create a positive mental attitude by recognizing you are getting more health out of your daily activities and more energy and time to enjoy the things you love.

We should always be looking at the different areas of our life and learning from others how to turn those moments into winning moments. These winning moments are not just to improve our lives, they are also to teach our friends and family a better way to live and enjoy life. If we can find activities that cause stress and reduce that stress on the body wherever possible by replacing it with a different way of doing that same activity, but now in a way that produces in the body strength, flexibility, endurance, and balance, is a major win for better health! Think of the impact that performing your daily activities multiple times in a day, 365 days a year, for years, has on your health. Are your daily activities being performed in a way that builds you up or breaks you down over time? I am on my never-ending quest to win as many moments as I can spiritually, mentally, and physically 24 hours a day, 7 days a week, 30 days a month, and 31 days on months that have 31 days, year after year.

Consistency is the key and the better we are able to consistently win moments in our day, the better opportunities we'll have available to live a healthy more active life.

Chapter 5

HOME REMEDIES

Here are some useful common home remedies. **This is NOT medical advice**, because I don't know what you are going through right now and more importantly why. These type of questions can only be answered by a thorough examination and proper diagnosis. **My first recommendation is to see the appropriate health care provider before practicing any of these home remedies.**

Cold Showers: Make sure this is safe for you and you have been cleared by your doctor. *Each day after your regular shower you can gradually begin to make the water a little colder and colder as your body begins to adapt to the cold water.* This is a process that requires time and consistency. Credit to Wim Hof for this method along with his breathing technique. Follow him on YouTube to learn more about the benefits and how to correctly apply his techniques, as well as what to look out for and who should avoid using this therapy. FIRST, CONSULT WITH YOUR DOCTOR AND WATCH THE VIDEO!

Deep Breathing: Deep breathing is a great tool to calm the body from stress, oxygenate your cells, release tight spots, and clear the mind. Be intentional about taking deep breaths when you are at home, work, and everywhere in between. When you find that you are back to breathing shallow, begin to breathe deeply again. When breathing deeply it will feel like you are filling your belly, chest, and even the top of your head with air. A powerful breathing technique is The Wim Hof Breathing Technique. You can learn about the many health benefits and find his tutorial on YouTube. Certain breathing techniques should not be done in the water, driving, or any environment that may be even remotely unsafe. There are many breathing techniques that you can use while relaxing your mind, find the one that is best for you.

Ice or Heat: Ice is the best thing to try first because of its' ability to reduce inflammation which is a common symptom of injury. The ice should be cold to the area, but it is important to not have it directly touch the skin. Use a towel to protect your skin. THESE INSTRUCTIONS ARE IMPORTANT...Only put ice on for 15 minutes at a time, then take the ice off for 15 minutes. This provides the greatest benefits that ice has to offer. If you know your body and it feels better with heat, then use the methods you have found to work best for you. Heat may benefit a person with chronic or muscular type pain. Be careful, when you first use heat it may feel relaxing, but when you take it off as the area cools the pain can increase. Be sure to protect your skin when applying heat as well. Some people like to alternate between ice and heat, always begin and end with ice. That's one of the reasons I always suggest starting with ice if you are unsure which to use. Once again your body knows best, so if you have a proven protocol that works best for you, that's what matters the most. I have a great video on ice and heat on YouTube https://youtu.be/k_fLmVCZ3IQ.

Muscle Cramps: Check your medication and hydration. First, check with your MD or pharmacist if you are on any medications. Cramps are a common side effect of many medications. *Next step would be hydration.* One good way to measure your water intake is that we should be drinking half our body weight in ounces each day. There are many fluids that cause dehydration, which means they cause us to lose water, like beverages with caffeine. If it is safe for you and you have checked with your MD and pharmacist, electrolytes help our cells better retain the water we drink, helping many people with cramps.

Prayer: Prayer is the most powerful tool I know. Stopping to invite and acknowledge God as the answer and joining him as he provides us with everything we need to do what he has called us to do.

Spinal Mobility and Power Posture: It is important for all spinal joints and discs to be in a posture of power and have a full range of motion to be healthy and protect the brain and nerve system. Spending time to get a chiropractic adjustment, putting the spine through different ranges of motion, and doing power posture work each day for the muscles, ligaments, and spine will improve every area of your life.

Stretching, Foam Roller, Trigger Stick: Muscle and Soft Tissue Therapy, is a great way to reduce stress and tight spots, while promoting health and healing in muscles, ligaments, tendons, and fascia. When stretching it is important to have a power posture and good form throughout the stretch. However, there comes a moment when you should be reading and responding to tight spots in your body. Making slight adjustments to stretch areas that feel tighter to help them relax. This makes the stretch more beneficial to you because it meets the needs of your body. Sometimes it includes relaxing parts of your body that aren't even included in the stretch like when you realize your mind is racing, you are clenching your teeth, your tongue is pressing against the roof of your mouth, or you thought you were relaxed until someone told you to relax your shoulders. In order to get to some deeper areas of tightness, it may require more time, like ten minutes or more of stretching in that one area. Take your time, try different stretches, learn more and more about your body each day, and you will get more and more from your stretching.

Water: Water is extremely important and should be the first thing you consume each and every day. Every part of your body needs it to perform their functions, it helps make muscles more flexible and pliable and detoxifies the body. The healthier the water the better job it can do in our body. Alkaline water is great. Check your local water supply, not all water is the same, even if it looks the same. Sometimes, I also add a couple tablespoons of apple cider vinegar to my water. You can read about the many benefits of apple cider vinegar at Mercola.com.

I don't expect everyone to take this information and utilize it all tomorrow. However, if you use it to change one area or win one moment in your life for the better, and you are able to do that with consistency, I know it will have the ability to have an amazing impact on your life.
God Bless

Thank you, God, for using me to write your book. All glory and honor to God my Lord and Savior. Thank you, Jesus, for saving me and the Holy Spirit for making a life possible I wasn't even capable of ever dreaming without you. Thank you for helping me to become less and for you to become more. Your ways are better and all your promises are true.

Chapter 6

MY STORY

I thought health was how I looked and felt, I loved to exercise, and worked at gyms. I would work out for hours each day and I loved to play basketball. I was exercising and eating right while at the same time I was destroying my spine, discs, and nerve system. You see, nobody told me how to take care of my spine. That's a big reason I want to make sure I help as many people as possible learn how to take care of their spine and teach it to their family and others. Because of the pain and discomfort I was in I went and had surgery because no one told me that there were any other options. Following the surgery, I had relief, but 2 years later I started to have the same pain again, fortunately, it was at that time that I learned about chiropractic care and how to care for my spine, discs, and nerve system as the foundation of health. Surgery had cut away the damage to my spine , but it did not remove what caused damage, which was a subluxation. Subluxation is a chiropractic term for a spinal joint that has lost motion and causes irritation to the spine, discs, and nerves. It is also the cause of spinal arthritis and many disc diseases, like degenerative disc disease. Once I started caring for the subluxation with a chiropractic adjustment schedule my health has been improving ever since. Each day I focus on the best ways to perform everything I do, even the littlest things, in a way that continually improves health, especially the health of my spine. This book is what I have learned from more than 20 years of experience. Some of my first lessons were how to live with excruciating pain, which lead me to learn about the power of chiropractic care and winning moments. Now, I've learned how to live a healthier more active life without pain, beyond exercise, stretching, and eating healthy. The same principles I have learned and used to get out of pain, I have found to be the same principles that allow my health to continue to improve each day.

Pain is a great teacher, guiding us towards better health, and a better way to perform the activities we perform each day. Pain has taught me a healthy way to do everything. Pain has taught me how to sleep, brush my teeth, shave, get dressed, tie my shoes, sneeze, cough, clean the house, get in the car, drive, get chiropractic adjustments, do soft tissue work, stretch, exercise, rest, keep a power posture, invest in my health every day...everything. It even gave me a purpose, career, and understanding of what people are experiencing, so I can better help them by improving their health with chiropractic care.

You may not need sleep, rest, water, good nutrition, strength, flexibility, endurance, balance, good posture, chiropractic care, soft tissue work, massage, acupuncture, physical therapy, yoga, dental work, yearly exams, blood work...to feel good, but your body needs them to be healthy.

I want to thank Jennifer, my wife, and daughter, Makenzie. We have things we love to do together and watching me obsess about being healthy may not be one of them, but you created the space for me to be me, so I say...THANK YOU!

Thank you to my parents... true fitness fanatics...I have many great memories of going to gyms, playing basketball, racquetball, doing aerobics, taking bike rides, runs, long hikes, and walks together. You guys are still going strong, I'm so glad we have a legacy of fitness to share with each other, and the time and quality of life, treasures, that those efforts have produced for us.

To my friends, we were so fortunate to grow up in a time that had walking(Chris), bikes, and skateboards (Dave) as modes of transportation.

Once we arrived at our destination, we would play basketball, football, baseball, lift weights(Justin and Phil)...and head back home, with amazing conversations and laughter all along the way.

Chapter 7

QUOTITORIUM

Health is like a bank account, you are either investing in your health, so you have plenty to spend on an active life, you have just enough and you feel problems when the account gets low, or you are suffering because you have not invested in yourself, you are spending like crazy, and the mental, physical, chemical, and emotional stresses of life, have robbed you of having the opportunity to enjoy a healthy active life.

Each day you are managing your health account by either building it up, which takes work and focus each day to take care of yourself or what commonly can happen is stress can combine with excuses about time, like you are too busy, I'm taking care of everyone else, I don't feel like it and little by little you are losing your health and the freedom and enjoyment that accompany being healthy.

People don't just wake up one morning feeling how they do, it is the result of the choices they make each day.

No matter what a person's health status is, they will always be a healthier version of themselves, when they invest in themselves each day.

It is very beneficial to do one or two stretches for your tight spots many times a day, in addition to the longer stretching you do once or twice a day.

3 Steps to Recovery from Repetitive Movement Injuries and how to avoid Injury all together. One is to ELIMINATE or minimize stress, by awareness, power posture, and muscle engagement...WINNING MOMENTS. Two CONCENTRATE on the body part involved to provide it what it is screaming out for...healing, with ice, stretching, and proper rest. The third is ACTIVATE, each day, over time, invest in that body part to make it many times stronger and more flexible than what any job or task will require.

Find a place to keep all your thoughts and lists. Once your mind knows your thoughts and lists are in a safe place, you will be able to think about other things, be more creative, enjoy being present, rest your mind or not think at all, enjoy a song on the radio, notice a beautiful tree you never saw before...You will ultimately perform better throughout your day, have more mental energy and focus, stress and worry less about trying to remember everything you need to do while making room for new thoughts. It also builds confidence seeing things get checked off your list, or if you need, you can just carry them over to the next day. Don't let what you didn't get done be your mental focus, it does not serve your greater self in any positive way.

The body is highly intelligent and makes very few mistakes, stiffness, tightness, and pain are to guide us to better health. These are cues that we are either missing something, not doing enough of something or haven't done something long enough, need to learn smarter ways of doing things, or have not given the body enough rest. When we find the right combination to help ourselves, the body will respond with better health. When we put our hand on the stove, the problem is the fire, not the pain. The pain causes us to minimize the damage and gets us to do what is best, get our hand off the stove, which gives the body what it requires to remove the stress and promote what's necessary for healing. Our body has always been designed to protect and repair itself, however, it does it better when we are not in our own way, treating symptoms and not taking care of the cause of the symptoms.

The heavier the object is that we are asking a muscle to move, the shorter the range of motion we should use moving that object.

The deeper the stretches we perform, the slower coming out of that stretch.

One chiropractic adjustment is good for the spine, but the number of adjustments your spine needs to be healthy is even better

When you put more and more good habits together, like nutrition, rest, positive mental attitude, spine health, exercise, soft tissue work..., you will get exponentially more out of each individual habit, and experience better health as a result.

Exercise, stretching, spine, and soft tissue work can be used as a break or powerful addition to your day instead of a distraction or burdon.

A car lasts longer and runs better when we take care of it, however, we still need our dashboard and computer to alert us to problems we need to address. Our body is the same way, we need to take care of it every day, and our computer, brain, will use symptoms to alert us to problems or areas that require more attention. Our dashboard will even tell us when we find the right activities to meet the needs of our body by taking away symptoms.

When a chef puts in all the right ingredients, they still do a taste test to add what they need to get the recipe just right. We can do everything right and our body still needs minor adjustments and additional attention to different areas to get through problems that arise or to take our health to the next level.

There are 656 muscles in the body, each person usually has 3-5 muscles that are causing them the most trouble. Stretching muscles, especially your trouble spots, 30-60 seconds a day, just 5 minutes a week, will produce incredible results. Consistency with stretching is what your muscles need and is the key to experiencing fewer problems and a more active life.

CONCORDANCE

Winning Moments in Alphabetical order...

B:
Backpacks
Balance
Bathroom/Toilet/Shower/Tub
Bed/Before Bed/Getting up from Bed
Breathing

C:
Car
Chiropractic Adjustment
Computer/Desk
Core
Cough
Cues

D:
Doors (Opening)
Dressed

E:
End of Day Routine
Endurance
Exercise

F:
Fascia
Feet Health

Finish your Day Strong
Flexibility

G:
Getting out of Bed
Getting Ready for the Day

H:
Hand Health
Hard Tissue
Healthy Habits
Home Design
Home Remedies

L:
Lift
Lunch/Breaks/Free Time

M:
Mattress and Pillow
Meditation

O:
Orthotics

P:
Physical Work
Pocketbooks
Posture
Prayer

R:
Relax Strong

S:
Shoes
Shovel
Sitting
Sleeping
Sneezing
Soft Tissue
Stay at Home Parent
Strength
Stress
Stretching
Sweep
Swim

T:
Time Management
Training/Exercise

W:
Wallets
Weekly Routine
Work Design

...MORE IN THE BOOK THAN ON THE LIST!!!